An Emotional Journey

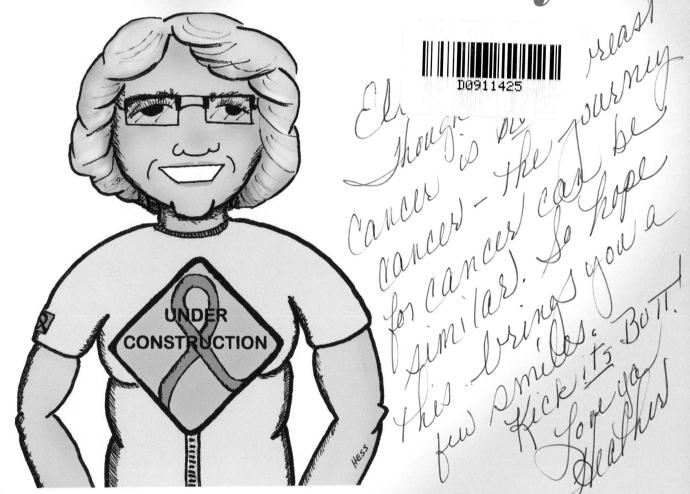

Humor AND *Hope* THROUGH BREAST CANCER

Heather Fiorentino

ISBN 978-1-64559-201-3 (Paperback)
ISBN 978-1-64559-202-0 (Digital)

First Edition

Covenant Books, Inc.
11661 Hwy 707
Murrells Inlet, SC 29576
www.covenantbooks.com

A portion of the proceeds from the sale of this book will be donated to help people with cancer.
Thank you so much for your support!

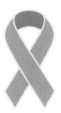

This book is dedicated to Marjorie Jeanne (Smith) Rose and Cheryl Klein.
Both courageous women encouraged me to draw cartoons to help others keep their sense of humor
during a frightening and difficult time as they battled cancer. Each lady spoke of the need to keep
a strong sense of humor as a part of the cure.

Note: *Marjorie was known to many as Maggie Rose, and to me, she was Mama. I love you and miss you, Mama!*

Acknowledgments

To all the brave women and men who kept their sense of humor and shared their stories with me during their battles with cancer, thank you.

With an overwhelming heart filled with love and appreciation, to my family and friends who took care of me, prayed for me, and helped to keep my spirits high with laughter while I fought my own personal battle with breast cancer, I offer each of you my sincere gratitude! It was many of your comments that gave me great material to work with for these cartoons. And it was your love and support which lifted me through my own low moments.

A special thank you to Jackie "Bever" Balogh for editing the cartoons throughout their development. Also, thank you to all the ladies and survivors for proofreading this book. To my nephew Chris Rose, a loving thank you for always being there for me and sharing your skills and talents to improve this project.

Each cancer patient who earns the title "Survivor" realizes it is due to the people surrounding him/her: family, friends, doctors, nurses, techs, staff, and God (*not necessarily in that order!*).

Thank you!

I would be remiss if I did not mention my husband, Joe, and daughter, Jenn, who were with me daily on my journey. I know they were secretly worried, yet they kept me laughing as you will see in the cartoons. They helped me to see humor in some emotional times. Thank you for putting up with my "cartoon-making mess" and reading each revision. It was your input and support for this book and me that made it possible to doodle my heart away. My desire is that this book can continue to spread the same laughter, hope, and support to others as you provided for me.

I love you both very much!

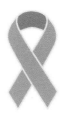

Table of Contents

PART 1: *Discovering Cancer* 1

Mammogram 4

The Cluster 5

Test Results 6

Waiting Room 7

YOU HAVE CANCER 8

Your Cancer Is 9

PART 2: *Prior to Surgery* **11**

Gender Hearing 14

New Uplifting Bra 15

Word Search 16

Bucket List 17

Lunch 18

Prayers Banging on the Gates of Heaven 19

Picture with the Girls 20

Kids Driving to the Doctor's Appointment 21

Minor Surgery 22

My Cup Runneth Over 23

PART 3: *Day of Surgery* **25**

Husband's Request 28

Needle Guided Surgery 29

Caring Husband 30

Are You Ready 31

Guardian Angels Assisting 32

PART 4: *After Surgery* **33**

I Am Good 36

Getting Prepared 37

Source of My Cure 38

Family Love 39

PART 5: *Radiation* **41**

Machine vs. Woman 44

Lightly Sautéed, Please 45

Grandma's Tattoos 46

Why Pink Stands for Breast Cancer 47

What's Burning? 48

My Lifesaver 49

Nite Light 50

Firm Up 51

Tissues 52

PART 6: *Chemo* **55**

Don't Be Afraid 58

College Prepared Me 59

Hairdresser 60

Lab Work 61

Pajama Party 62

Kneel for Strength 63

True Color 64

Puppy Hair 65

PART 7: *Some Good Thoughts* **67**

Happy Birthday 70

Double Breasted Jackets 71

Intentional Left Flat 72

We Need Some Clouds 73

HOPE 74

With CANcer, I CAN 75

First Syllable 76

Survivor 77

Introduction

In 1983, Marjorie J. Rose was battling breast cancer. She faced each day with a smile and a positive attitude. She made the best of each day and every moment.

Marjorie was my mother. Mama (as I called her) would share her funny stories of some of the obstacles that she faced through her battle. During her daily adventures of having cancer, she always found at least one humorous event to share with me. Since my father fought in three wars and served thirty-eight years in the army, Mama was happy her battle was at home with her family nearby and not in a foxhole on some "balmy island."

At the same time Mama was fighting breast cancer, a fellow teacher, Cheryl Klein, also started battling cancer. She too had the same positive outlook and a wonderful sense of humor.

Both ladies would tell me their tales of interactions and adventures throughout their fight with cancer. I would visualize the stories as cartoons in my mind. Then I would "doodle" some of the stories into cartoons.

Eventually, I combined my original cartoons into a small book, which I presented to Cheryl as a reminder of her spirit of hope. Unfortunately, I did not keep a copy.

There have been nine members of my family who have fought different types of cancers. So in my family it is said, "It is not if I get cancer, but when I get cancer." It is my belief Mama taught all of us how to face the fight with grace, a sense of humor, and a strong faith with a friendship with God. The humor assists to strengthen our hope and is used as a weapon to beat cancer. It is the job of all family members to see the positive moments and share in the laughter. The positive attitudes will boost everyone over the hurdles of the day. Everyone needs to pray for the one who is sick and for the family as a whole.

So fast-forward to December 19, 2013, after my six-month follow up mammogram, sitting in that fashionable paper gown, the radiologist stated, "This is not good. You need to see a surgeon." It was not the first time I had heard those words or seen that look, thinking, *One more scar to be added to the collection…my breasts are starting to look like a train yard with all the train tracks (scars).*

After the biopsy in January 2014 in the surgeon's office, I heard the words no one wants to hear: "YOU HAVE CANCER." Those words rang through the room until they stifled the air. It was amazing how easily those words roll off the doctor's lips as if saying, "Good morning."

The canals of my ears became clogged with those words. My brain became frozen, all unbeknownst to the doctor who continued talking. That day, I came home from the surgeon's office and started doodling my feelings and some memories of stories from family and friends. Over the next six months, the draft of this book was born.

There are some very talented artists and some individuals with God given skills in the realm of art. I am a "doodler." My doodles are good enough to express my message and share some humor. So the perspective may be off and the dimensions might not be accurate; therefore, I ask you to enjoy my ability of finding the humor within these serious situations.

This book is for you, the reader. We all have been touched by cancer, whether personally, or through a family member, or a friend. My wish is you will find the humor to help strengthen your hope and courage while realizing you are not alone during this journey. Other survivors have experienced the weakest moments you are feeling.

Find a survivor to talk to or contact a support group. I pray this book gives you some laughter, hope, and strength. If it touches your heart and strikes a funny bone while seeing yourself or a loved one in some of these situations, my mission is complete.

May God bless you and provide you courage and strength.

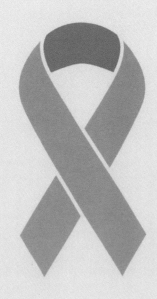

PART 1

Discovering Cancer

1

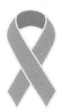

Each year, you go for annual tests that your doctors order, and it's just a matter of fact. It's September…time for a mammogram.

You do not think much about it until you receive a call to come in as soon as possible for the results. Then you learn you may need additional tests or a biopsy. Oh, how your heart sinks and time begins to move so slowly as you wait for those results.

Your worries begin to grow and time drags on. If you hear the words, "YOU HAVE CANCER," your world stops. Denial may arrive in your mind. But it doesn't matter, because you are numb, and the mind is stunned with the overwhelming news.

You have officially started on the journey…

Let's find some understanding and humor of your emotions on this journey…

Mammogram

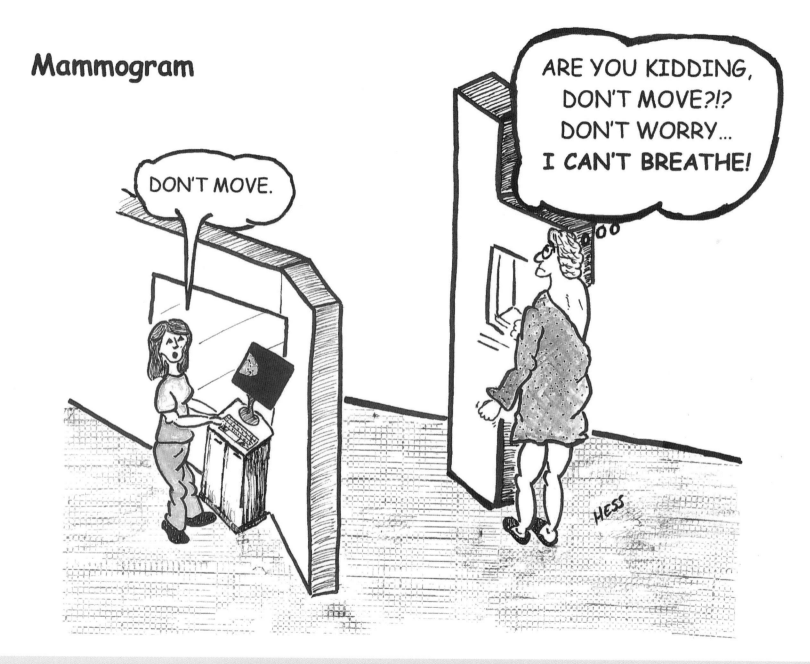

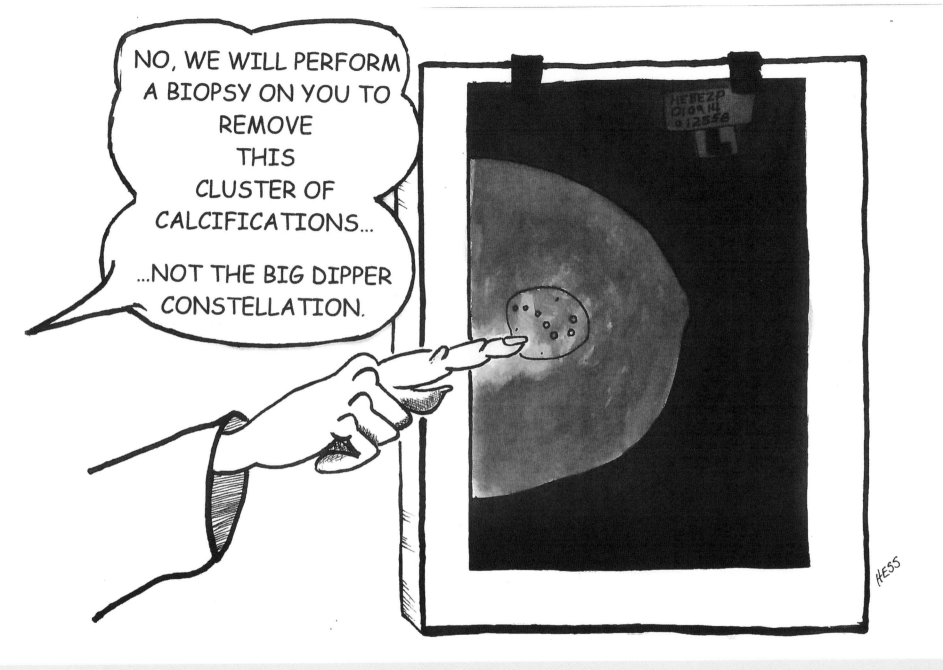

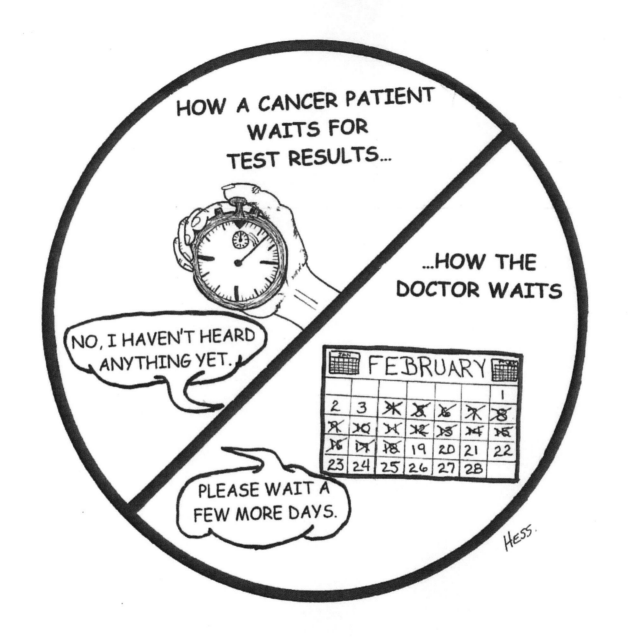

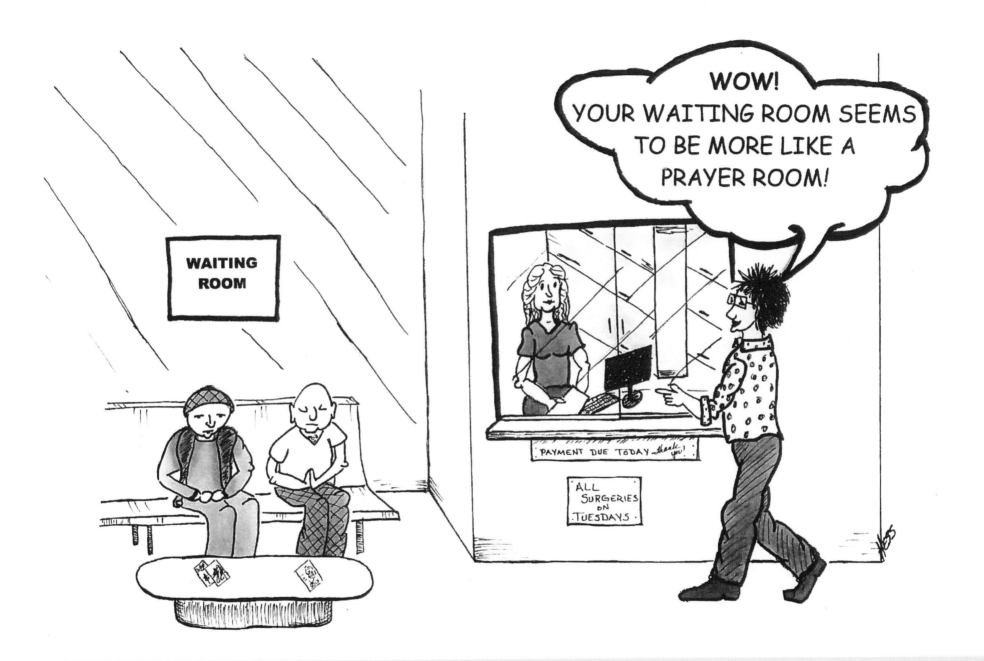

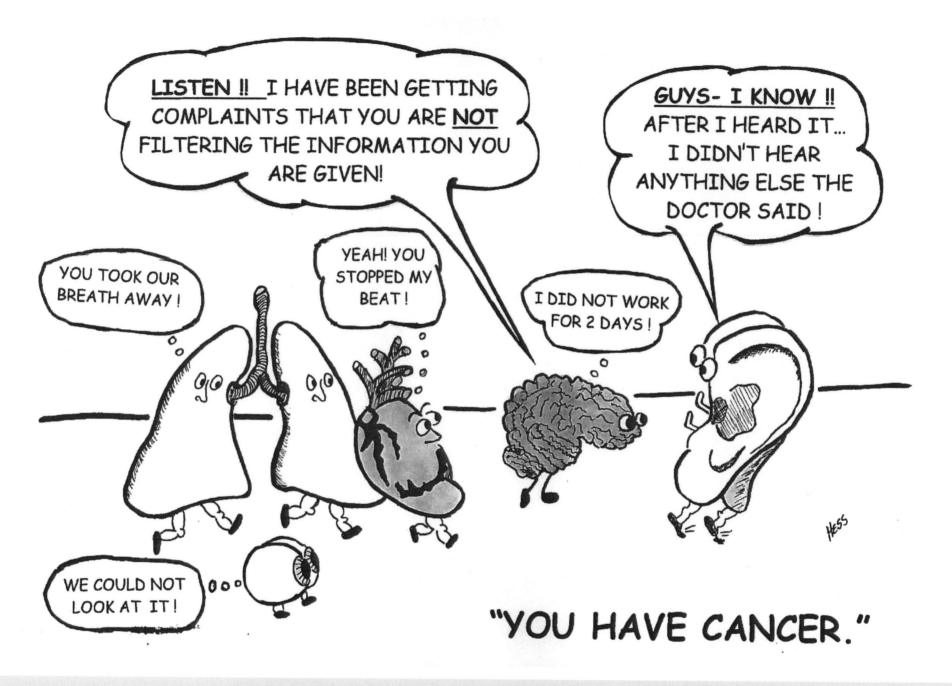

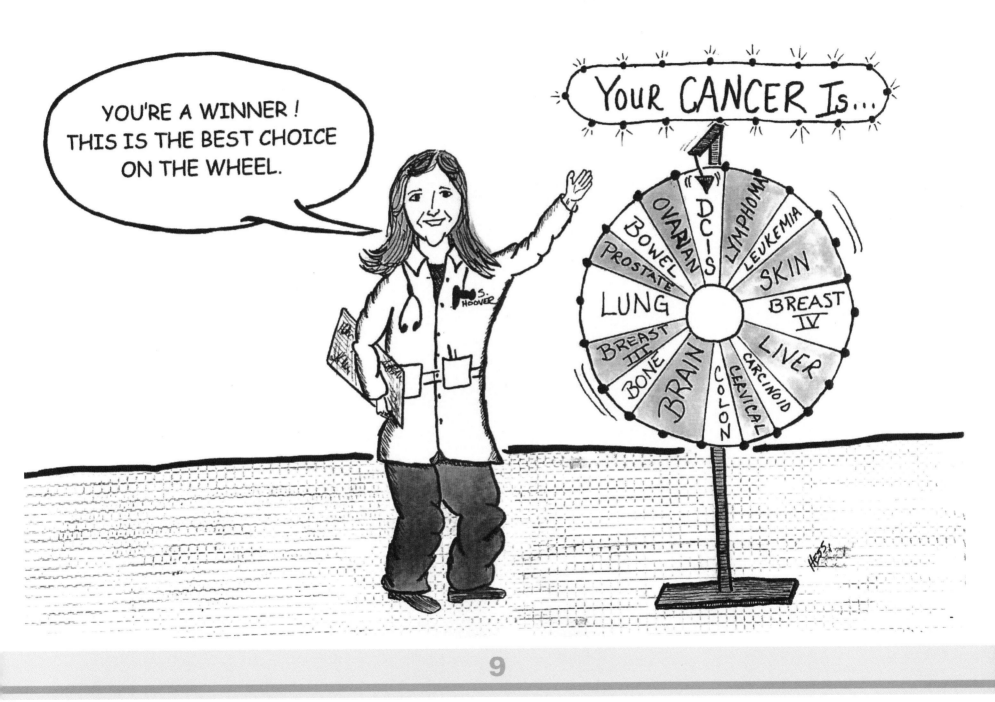

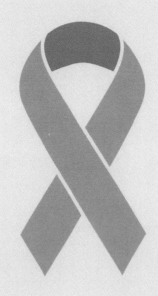

Part 2

Prior to Surgery

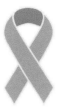

Now the numbness becomes reality. Choices have to be made—some by you, some by the doctors. You only have a few weeks or less to make decisions about your life on a subject you know nothing or very little about. The fear sets in, and conversations with God begin for you and your family. The family becomes closer, and the doctors' visits increase until a plan is prepared to meet your individual needs to fight the cancer with a victorious outcome.

Let's find some understanding and humor of your emotions on this journey...

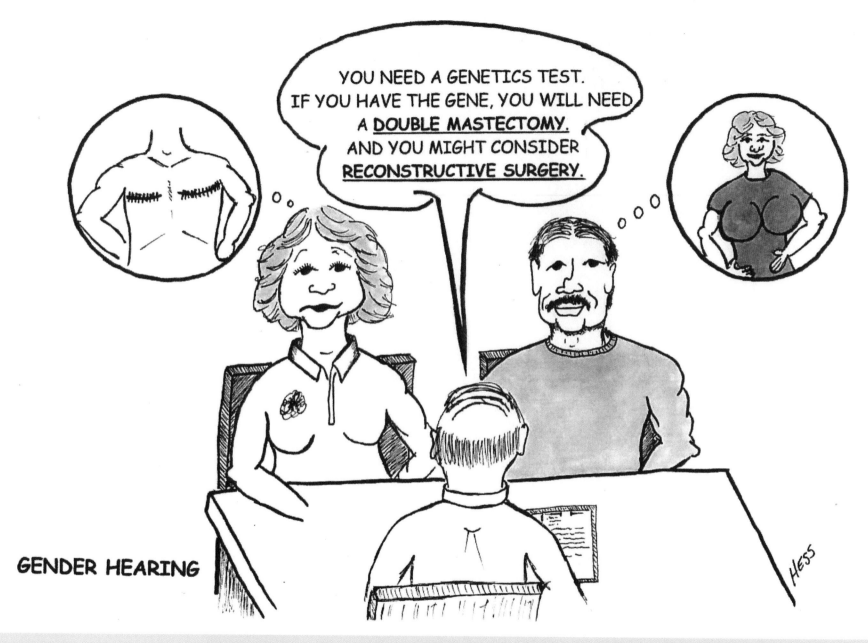

GENDER HEARING

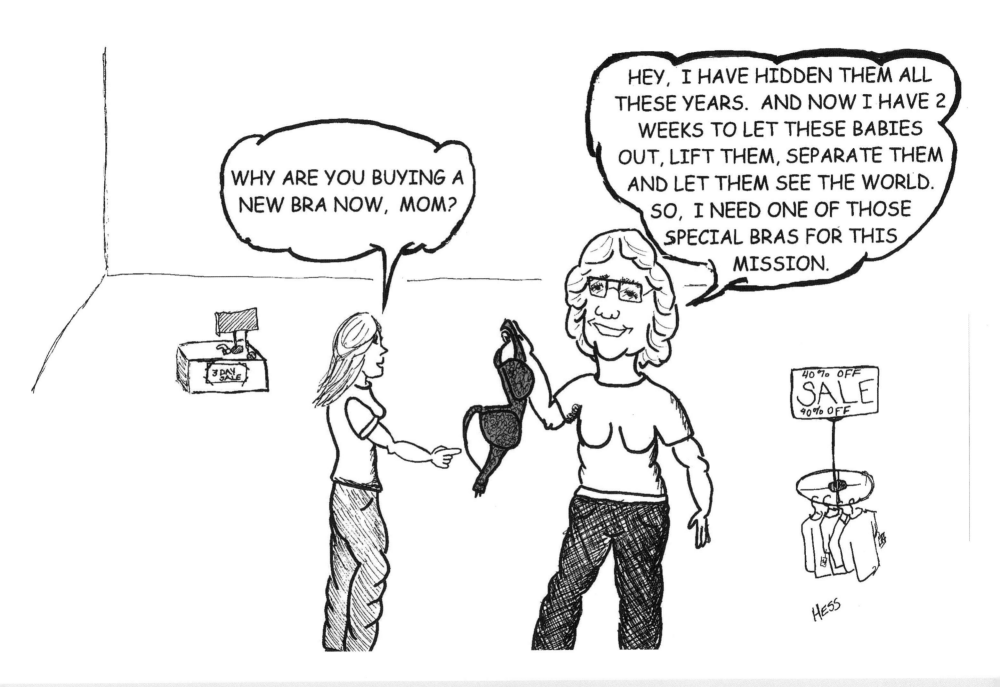

FIND THE BREAST

```
B O O B O S O M B O B B C H S
S R E S R O O H O O T E R S E
B T S C H E S T C H O O B O H
O T I C H E A T B O O B I E C
O M A M M E L S O O T I T I L
B T P M E L E N T I T S S B E
C H A T G A M E H E S T T O A
E T I T E A V M E L E I B O V
A O R I A S O G M K T T T A
V R I B N S C T I N N T I E G
M E M C O K T O R O O I R R É
M M E L O N S I L C C E S S I
G I R L E A V T S M K S S T T
G R I L G I R T L B E E O O B
T T H E S H E L F E R R E A V
I T H E L V V V F É S R O O V
B O O T I E A V B M E L V E B
```

FIND:

BREAST   HOOTERS   TITTIES

KNOCKERS   MELONS   TITS

BOOBIE   PAIR   TATAS

BOSOM   CLEAVAGE   CHEST

THE GIRLS   THE SHELF   BOOBS

*Answers
see page 78:*

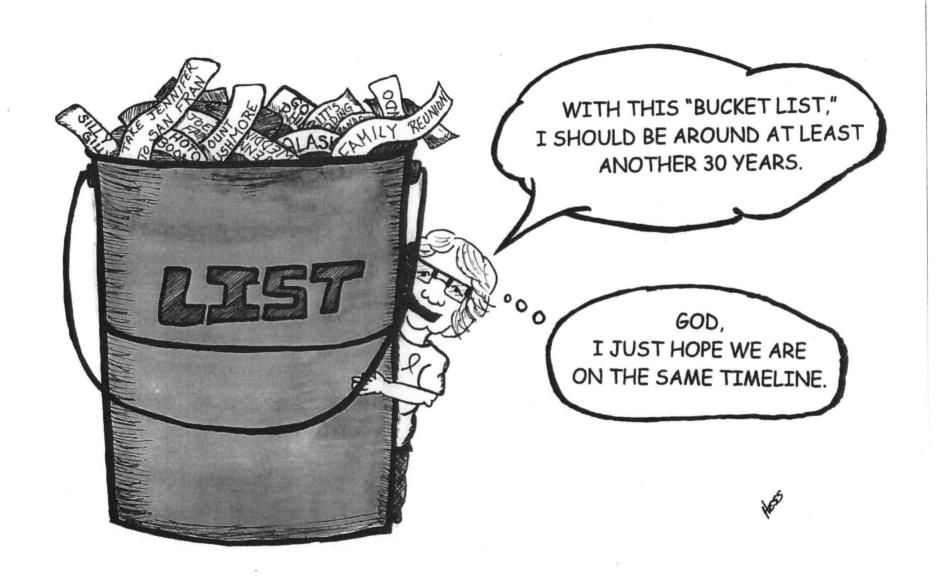

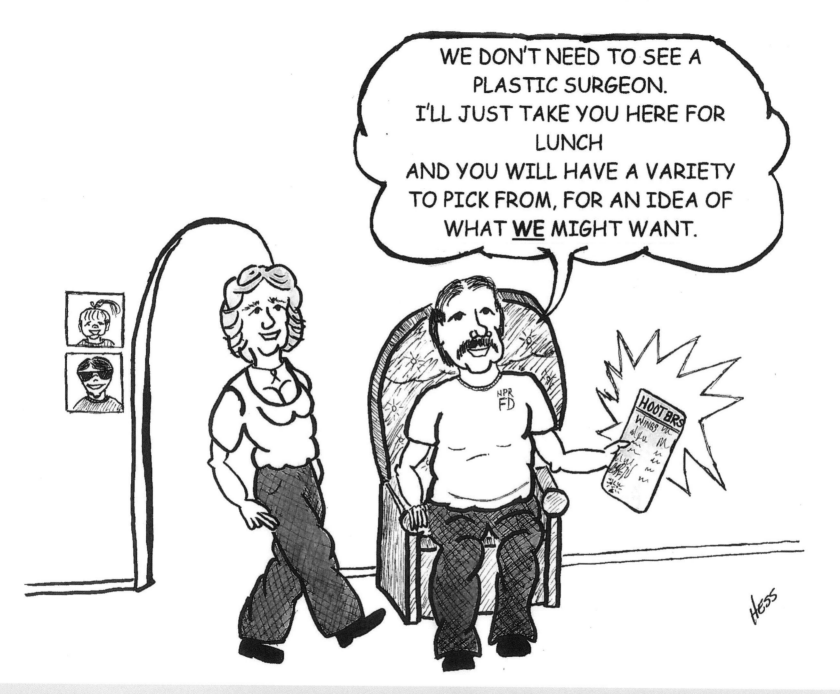

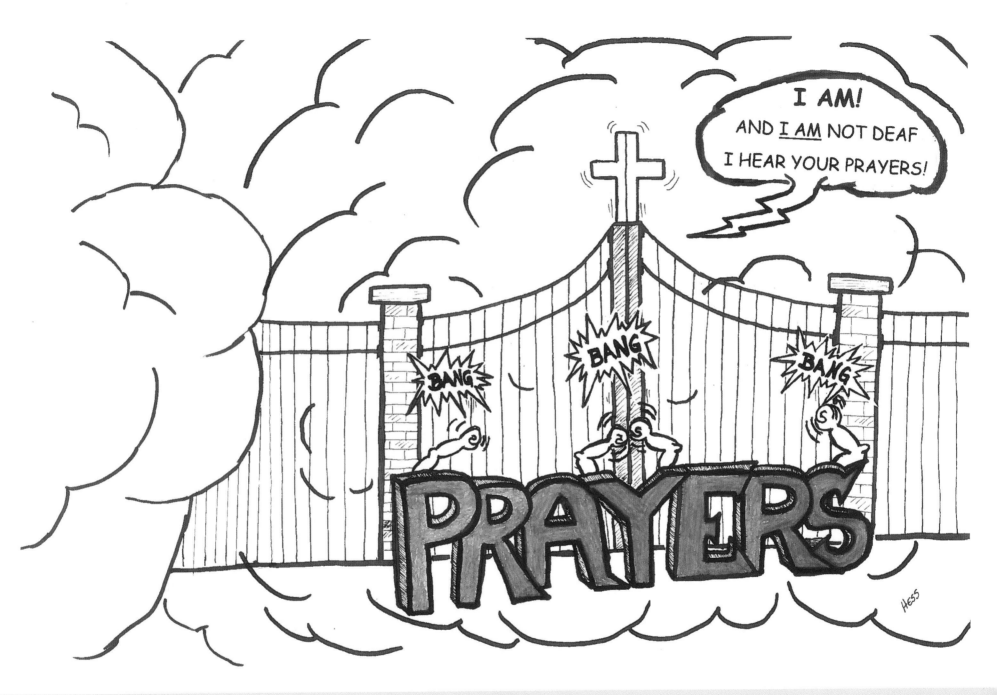

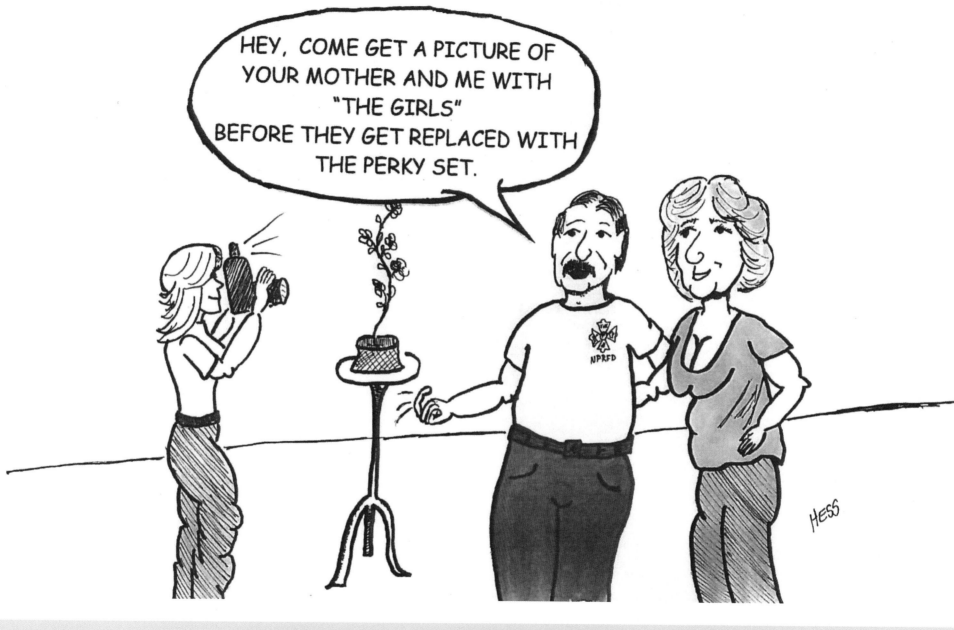

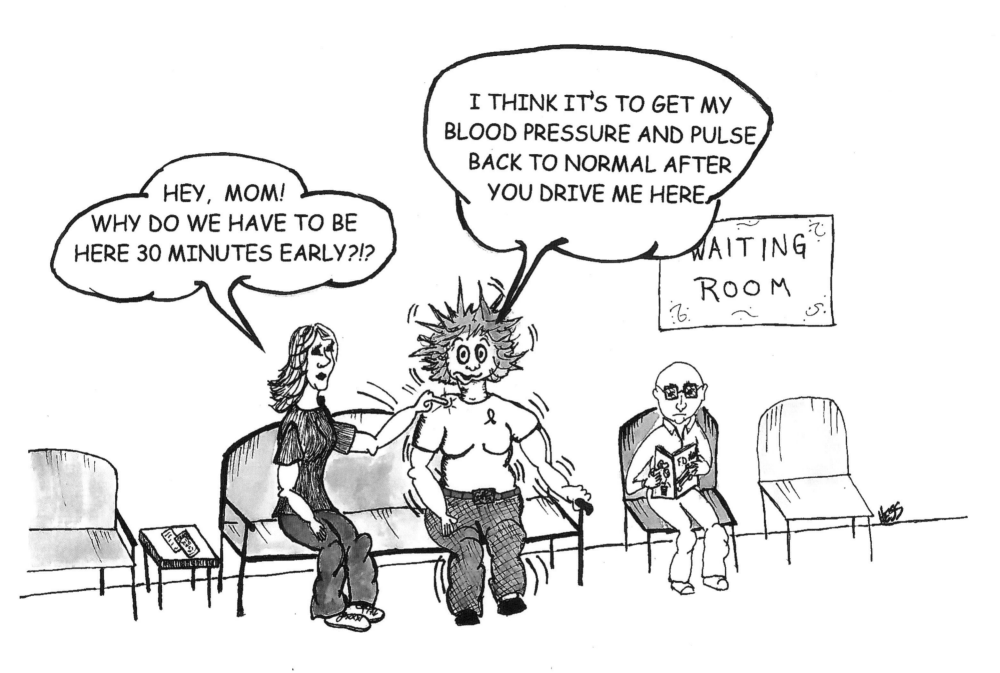

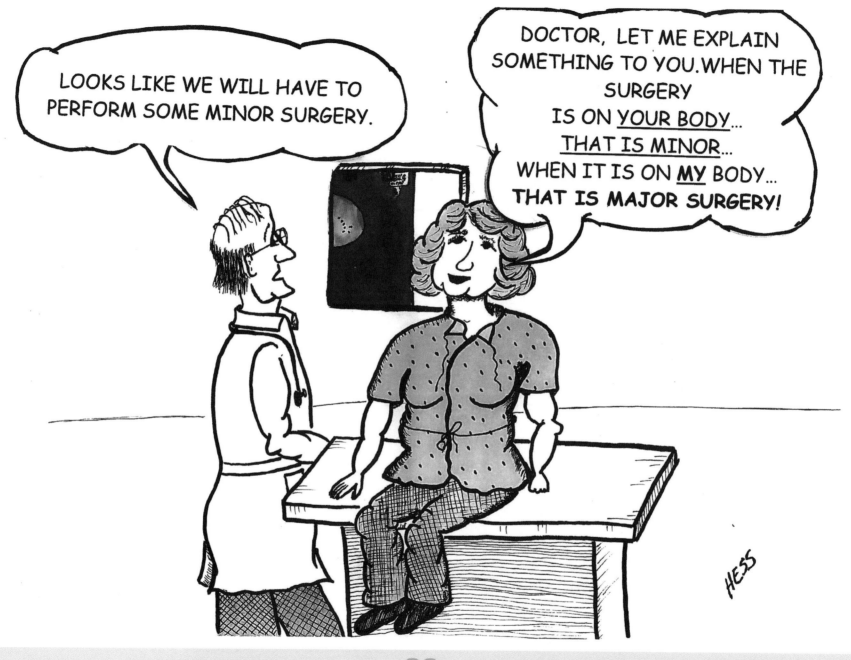

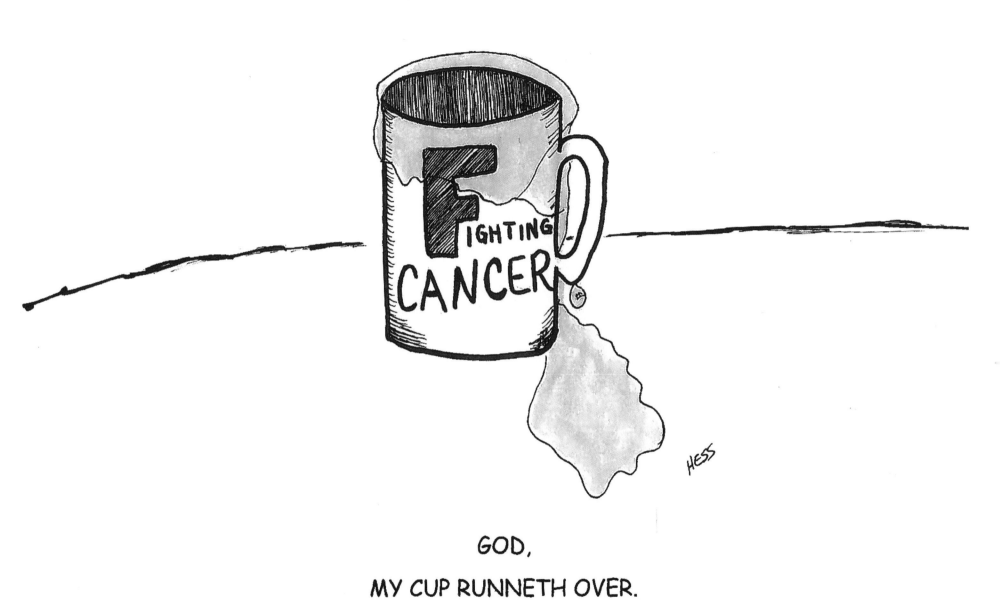

GOD,

MY CUP RUNNETH OVER.

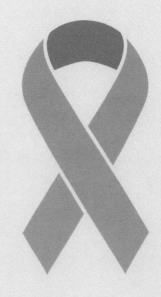

PART 3

Day of Surgery

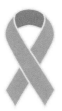

The day has arrived to remove the unwanted abnormal cells/tumor growing in you. First, marking the location of the cancer needs to be done to assist the doctor to remove the cancer.

Remember, your part of this day is easy; your family is in the waiting room, praying and making deals with God as each minute ticks away. Sometimes, no matter our age, we even wish to speak to our parents (whether they are with us or not) to find some comfort and protection. This is the first major step of your journey, although you feel like it has been forever to arrive at this point.

Let's find some understanding and humor of your emotions on this journey...

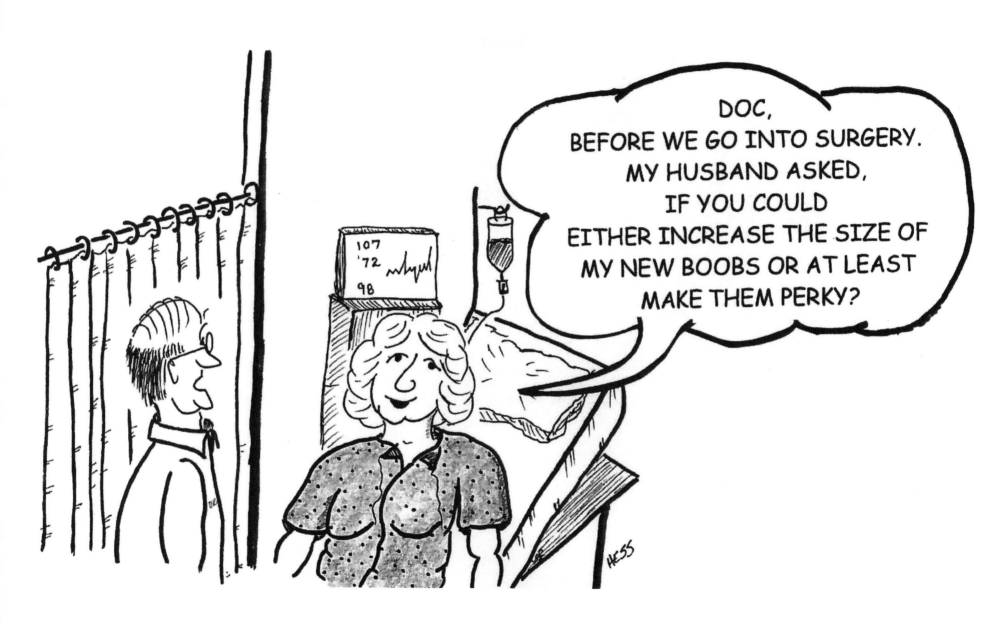

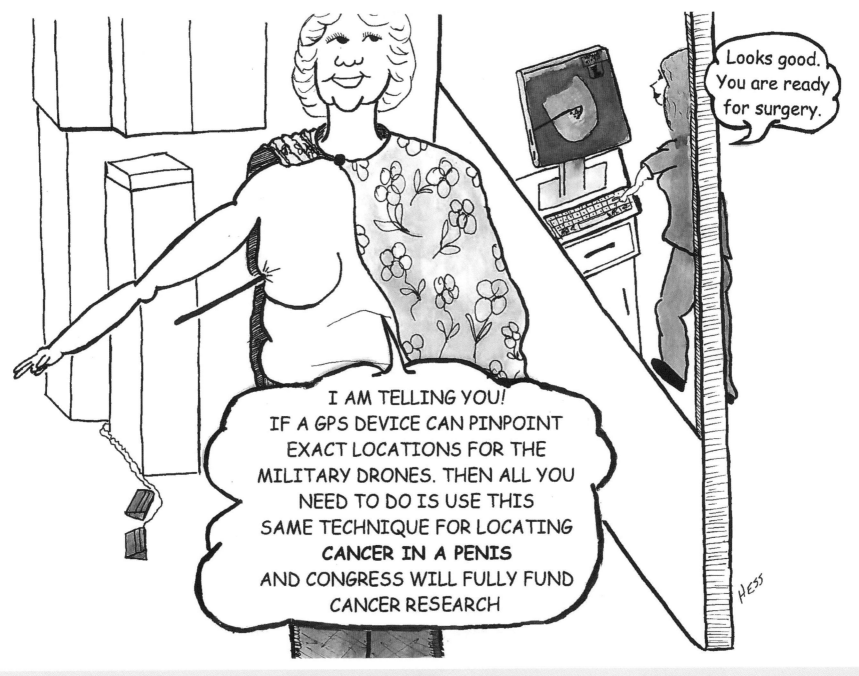

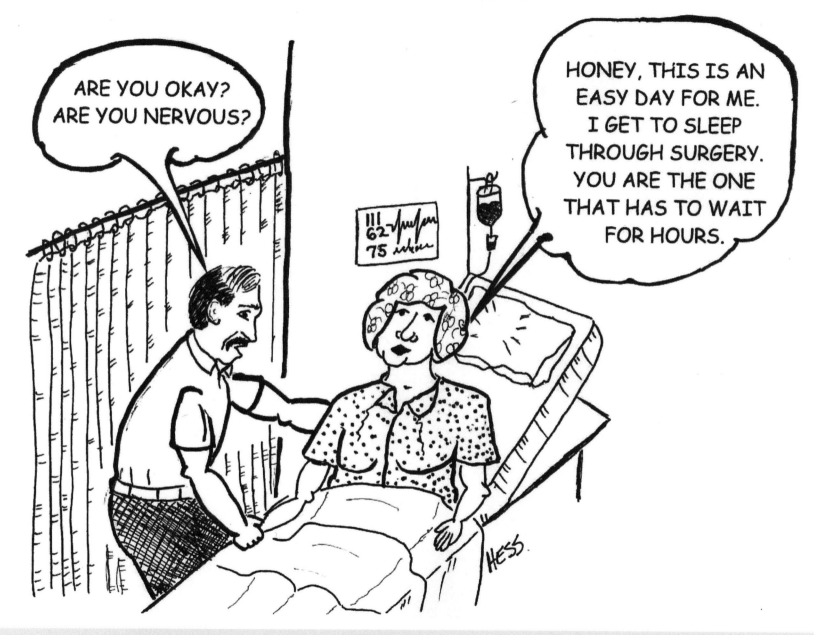

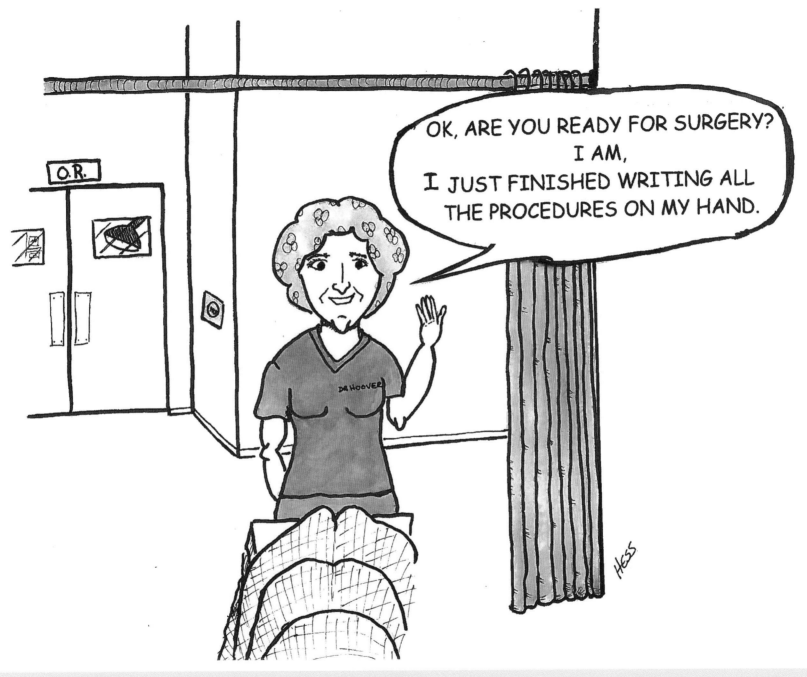

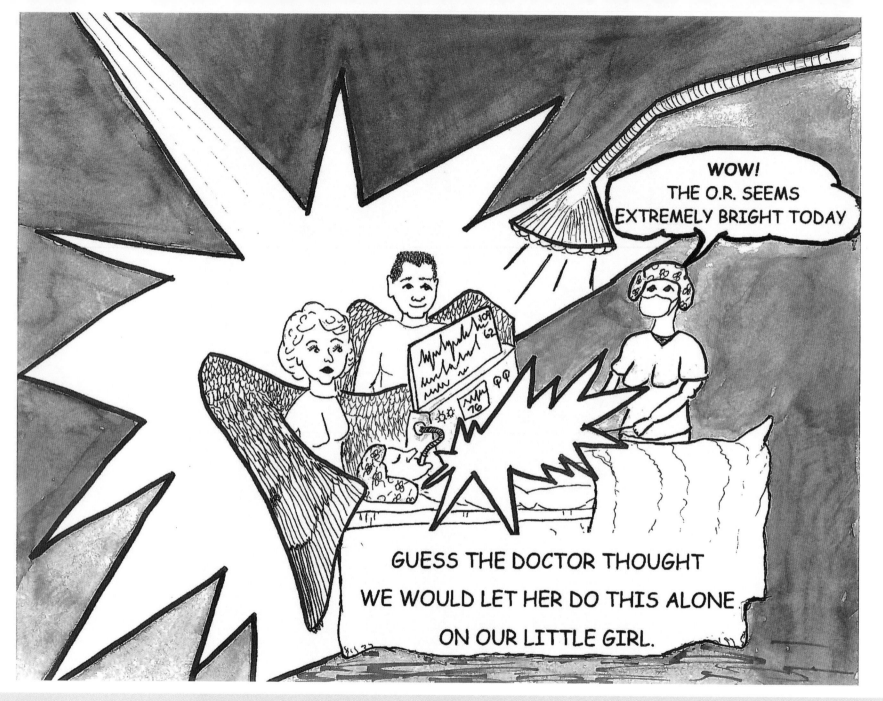

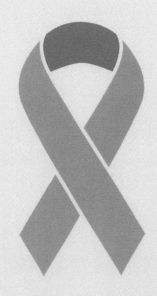

PART 4

After Surgery

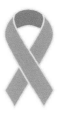

All margins are clean, so you can continue to heal and mentally prepare for the rest of the journey that you and the doctors have planned to prevent the abnormal cells to grow and/or multiply. You know that all or a major portion of the cancer is out. Yet, the fear grows that the cancer may come back or you fear the next few months with treatments ahead. If God was not on your speed dial before, He is now. You feel love from all those around you.

Let's find some understanding and humor of your emotions on this journey...

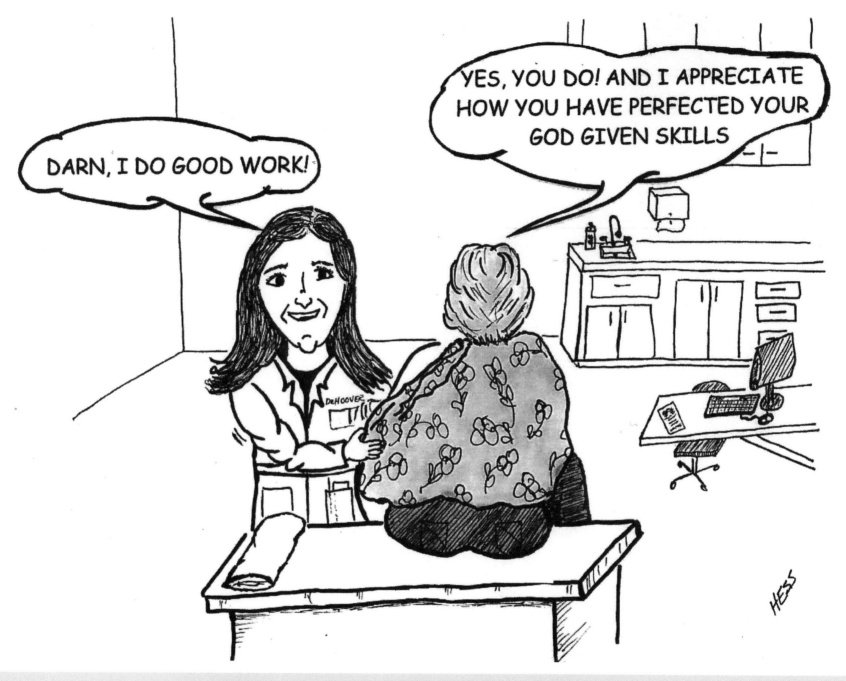

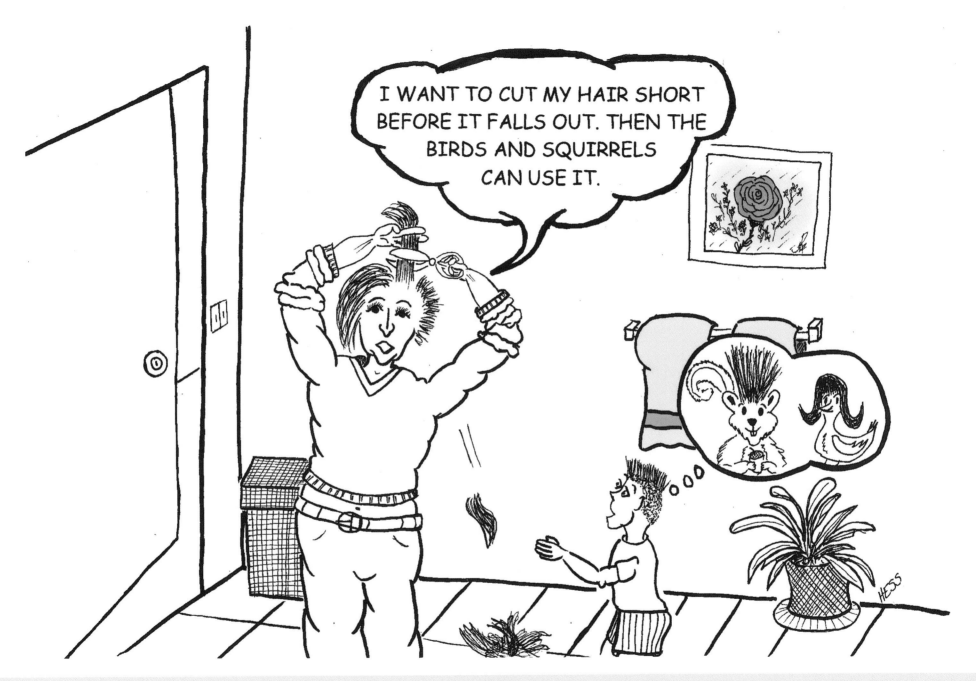

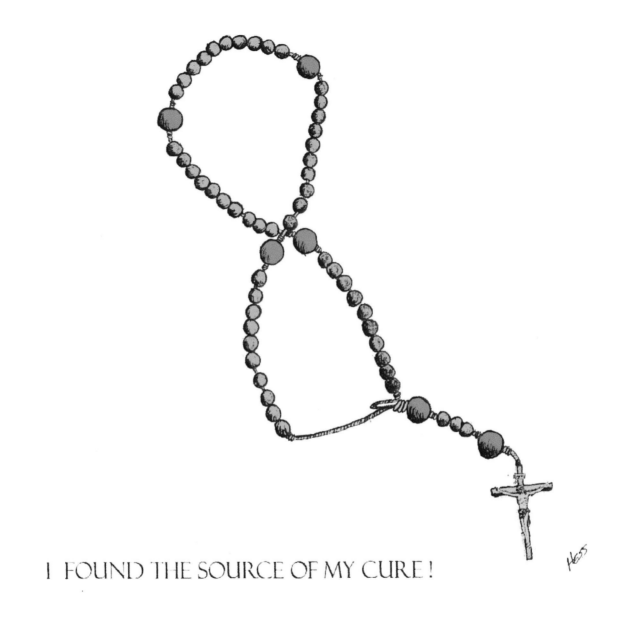

I FOUND THE SOURCE OF MY CURE!

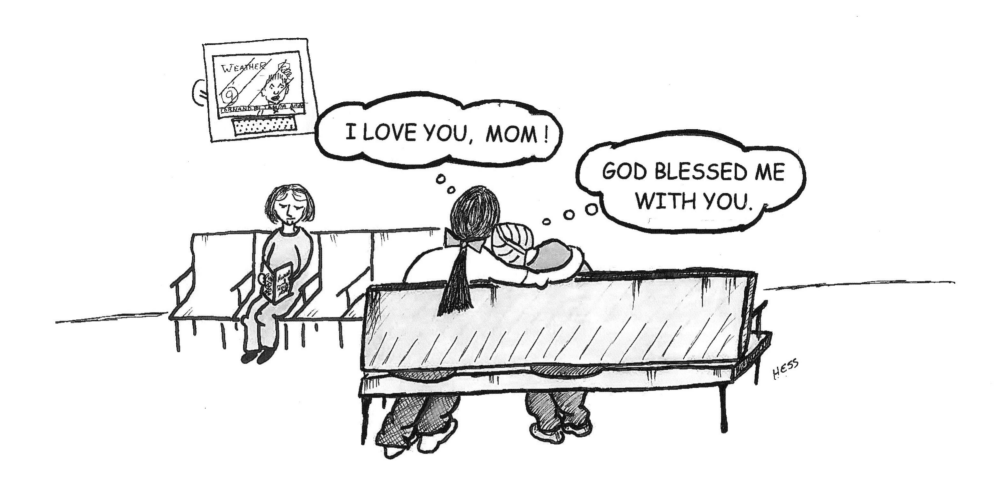

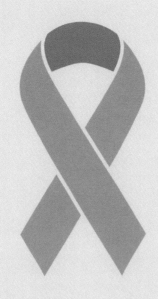

PART 5

Radiation

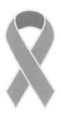

You are doing great, still moving forward. You have heard the words, "You Have Cancer," and you are still alive with a plan in place. The surgery is behind you; now for the start of your treatments.

You feel alone and scared. Next are the preparations—being tattooed to line up the radiation beam, and fitted for your cushion cast or the board with arm brackets. Whatever is used, it is not comfortable in that cold room with that huge machine shooting beams at you. Yet, you know the linear accelerator (also called a LINAC) is supposed to help save your life as it burns and tightens your skin.

The daily setup time for your treatment can take ten to fifteen minutes, and the treatment may last seconds (usually less than 120 seconds). Many people I know have used that time to pray. That was my time to study the machine so I could doodle it.

Let's find some understanding and humor of your emotions on this journey...

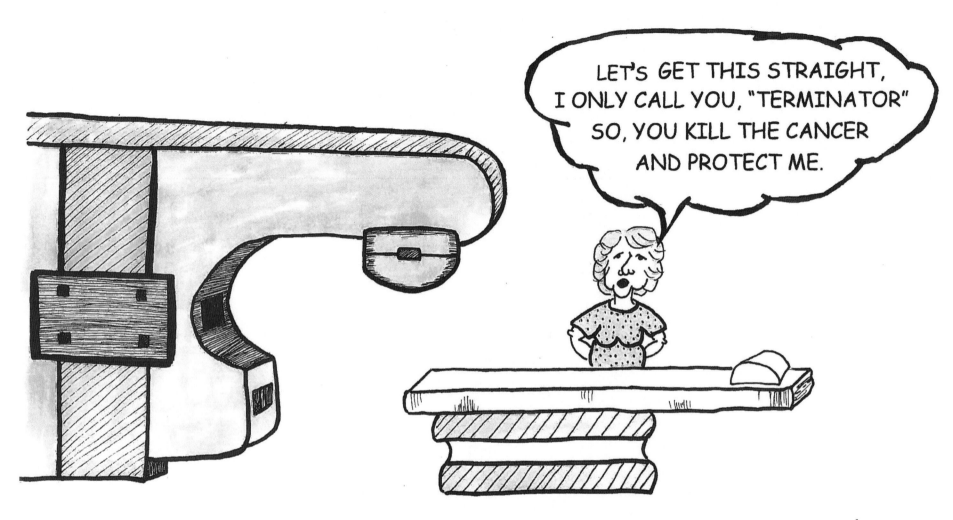

MACHINE-VS-WOMAN

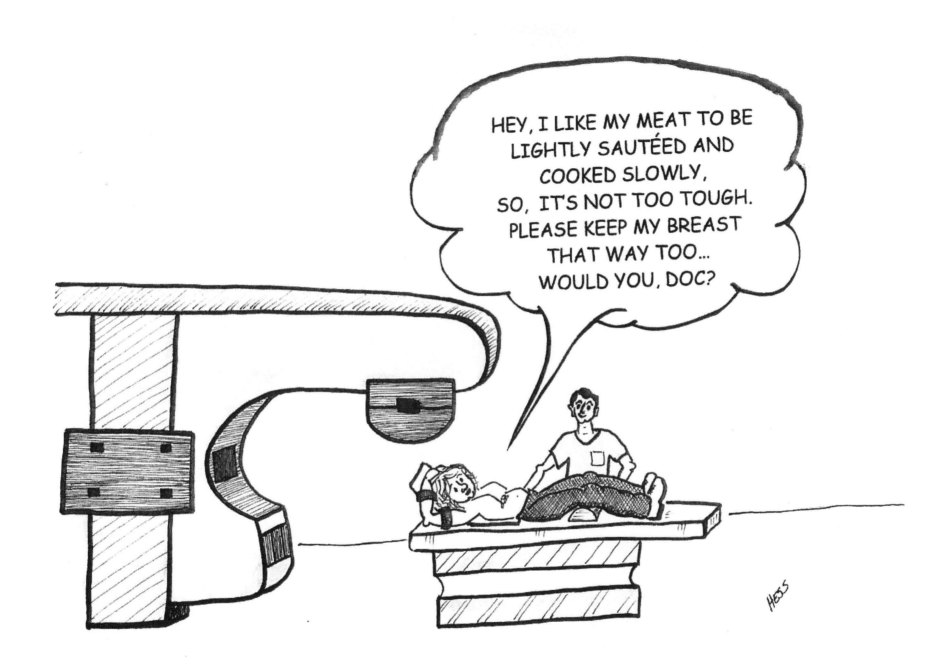

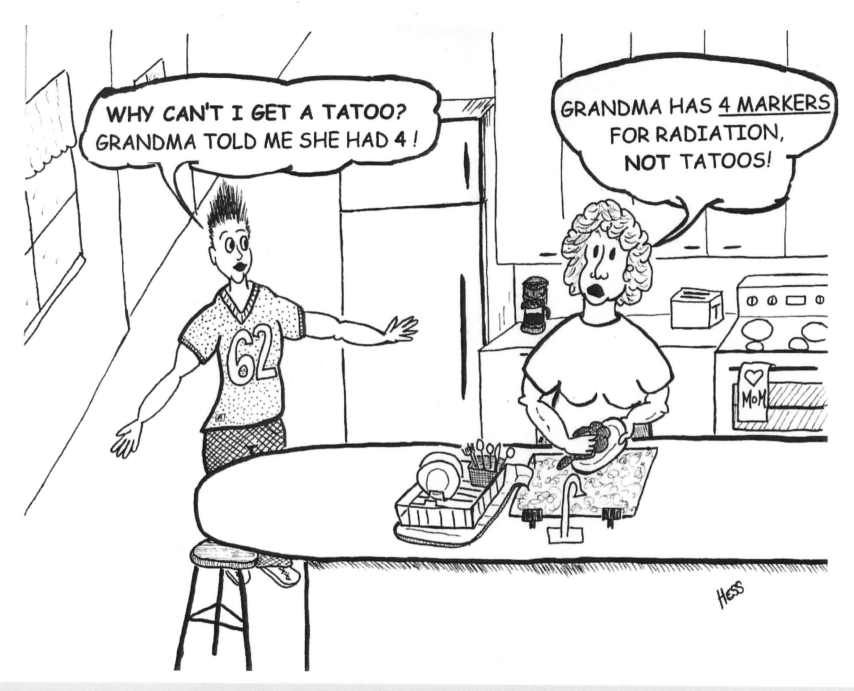

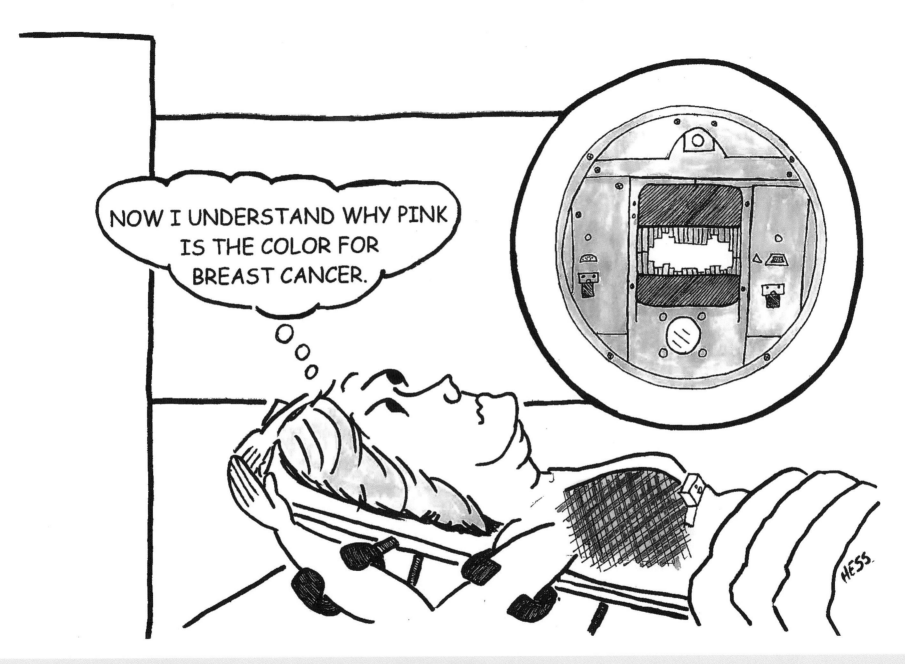

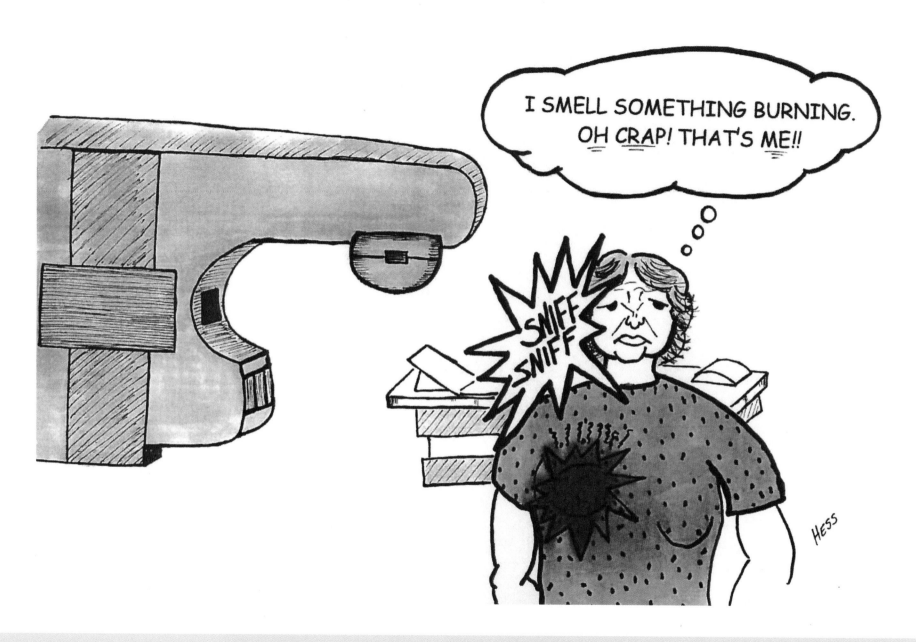

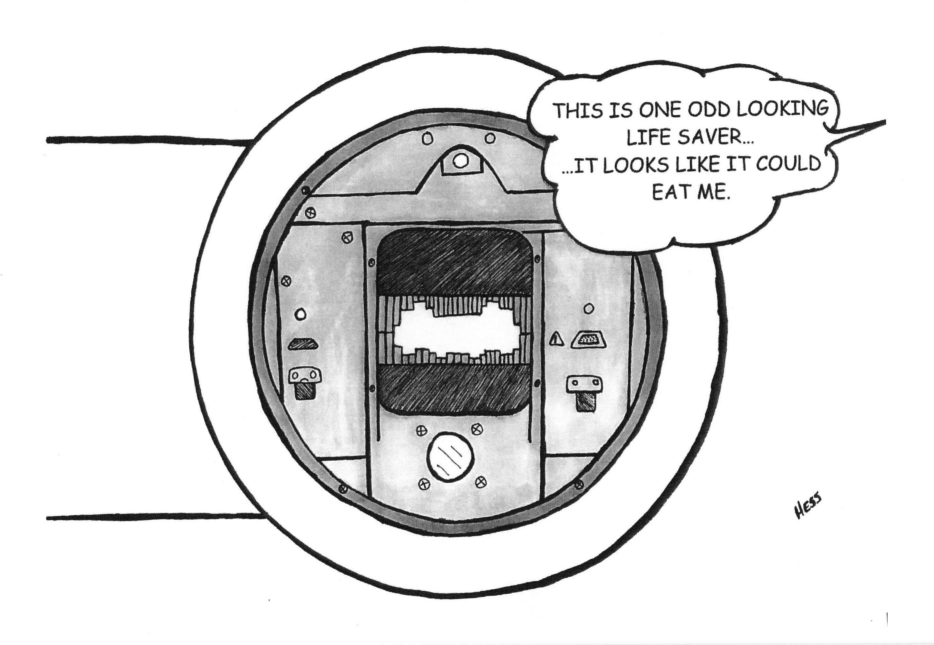

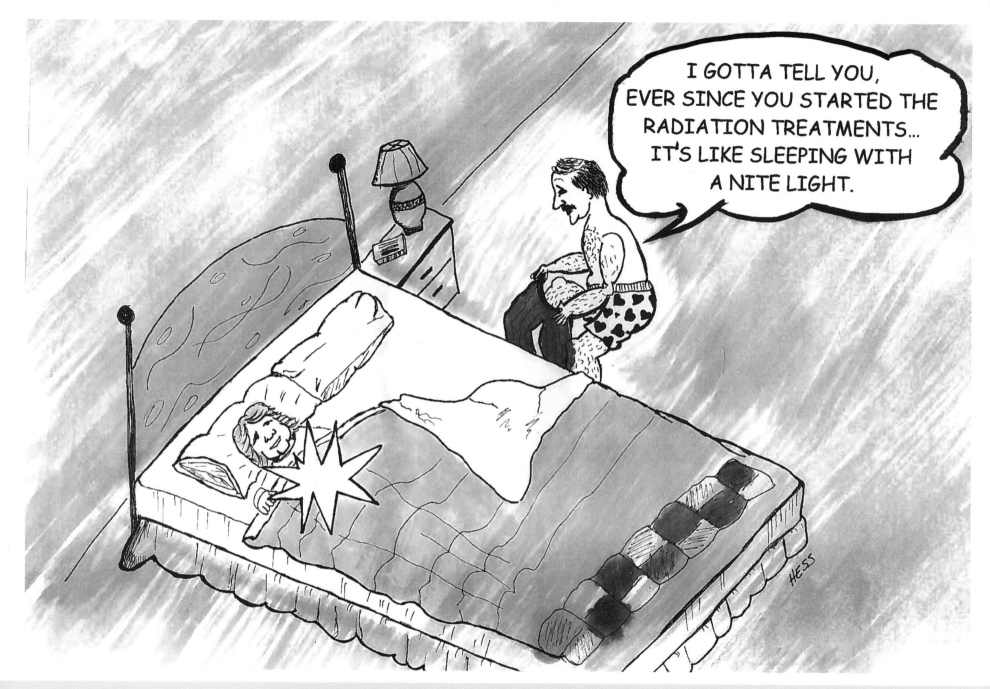

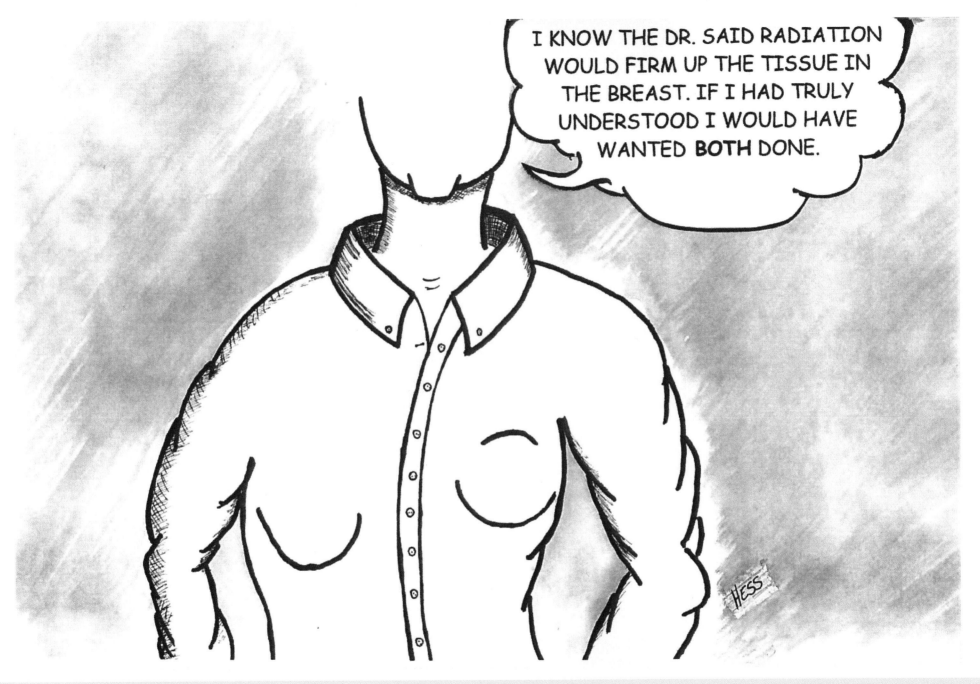

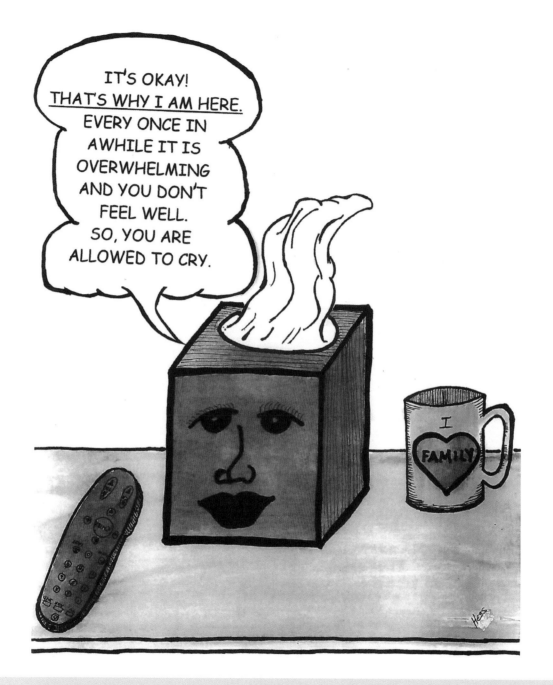

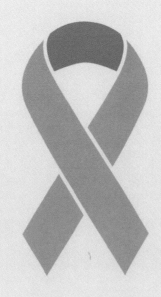

PART 6

Chemo

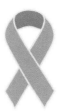

Have you realized you are not alone on this journey? Have you realized life and family are important, not the job or any other things that you may have thought important a year ago? You do make new friends at your clinics or with individuals who are survivors. People who understand the emotions you are feeling and who realize life and family are important, not the job or any other things that you may have thought important a year ago. We share encouragement with each other and may find humor that our outside friends may not understand; and we try to comfort one another as we sit and wait. Some people lose their hair, some lose weight, and no one loses hope or the light at the end of the tunnel…that is where we see our families cheering and waiting for us.

Let's find some understanding and humor of your emotions on this journey…

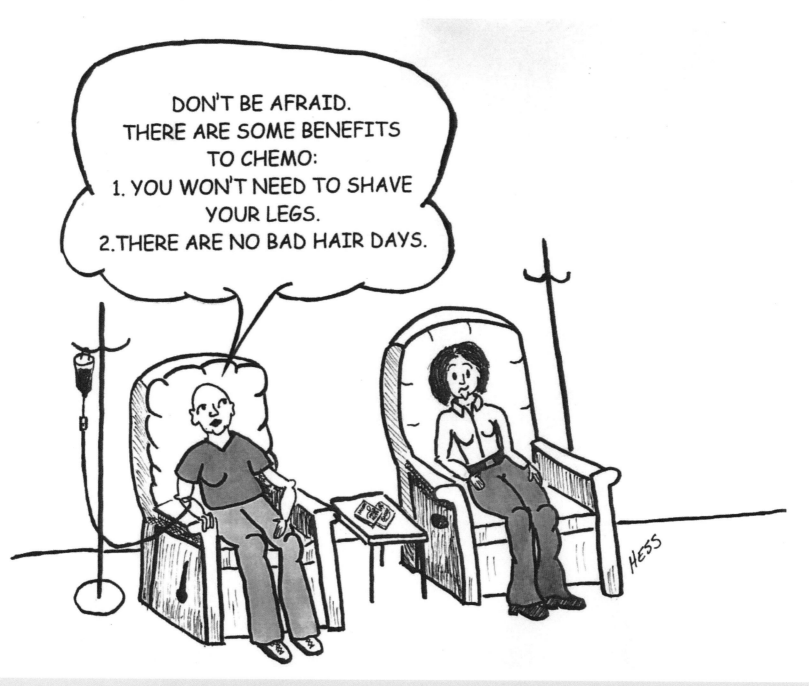

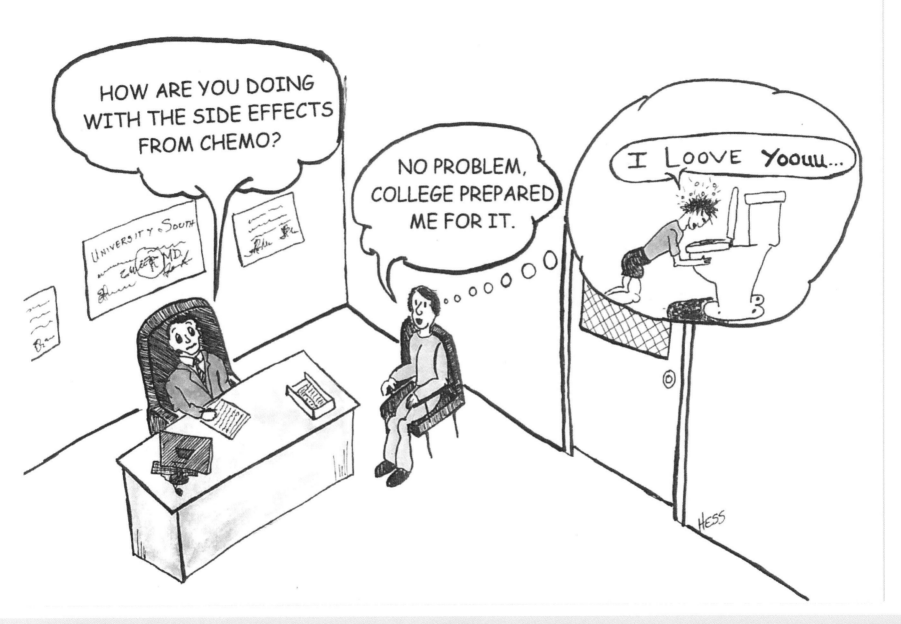

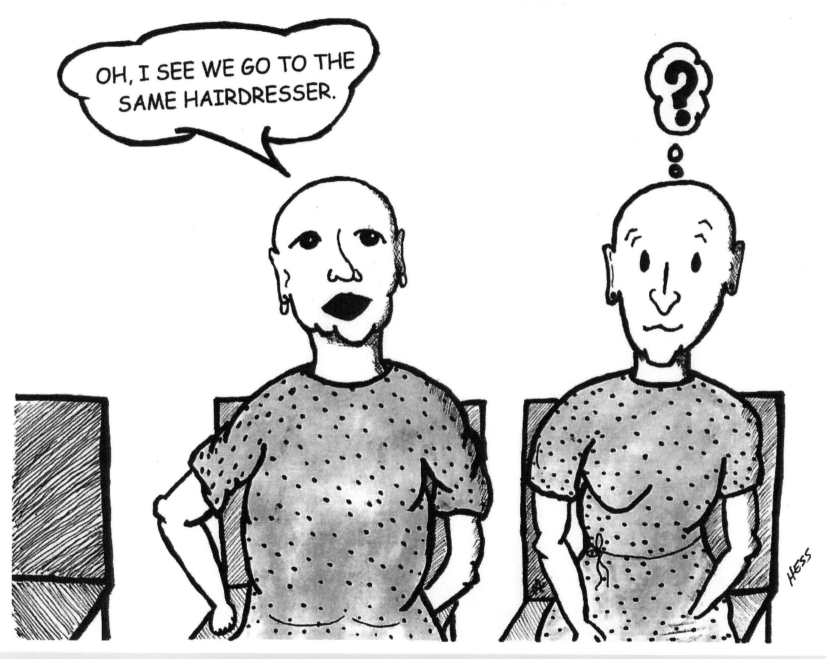

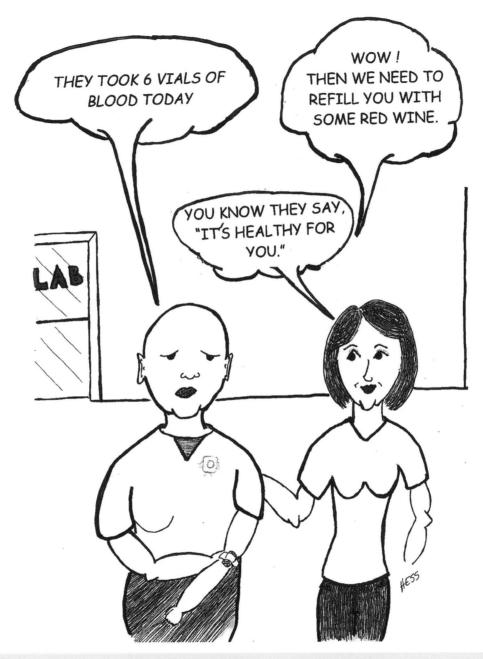

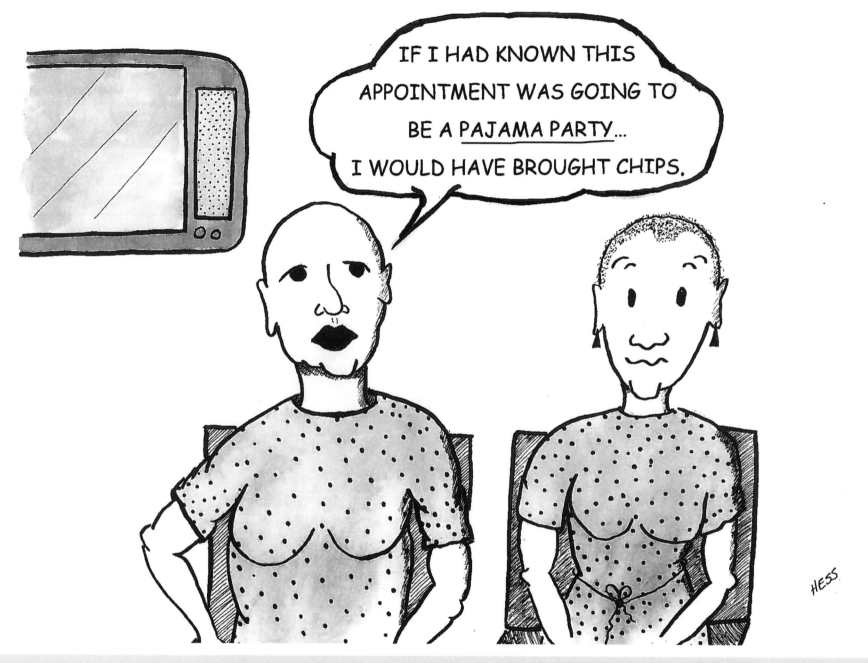

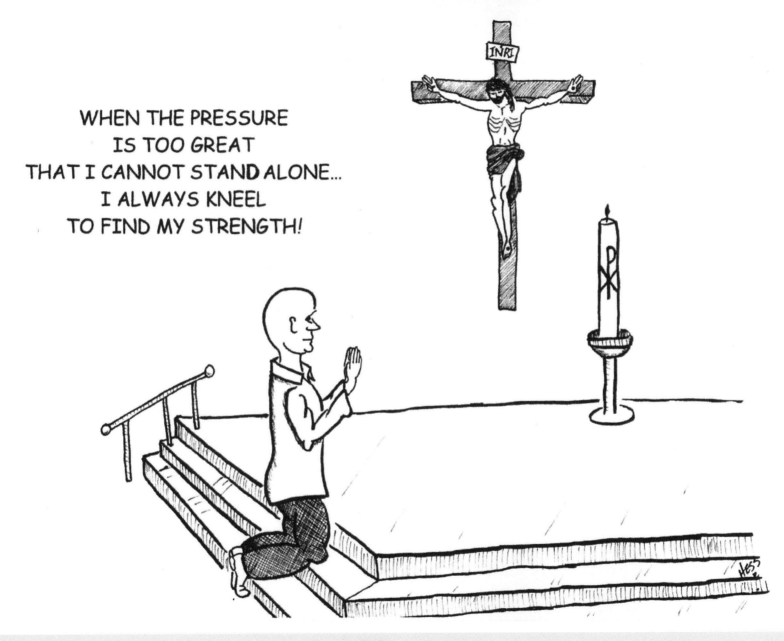

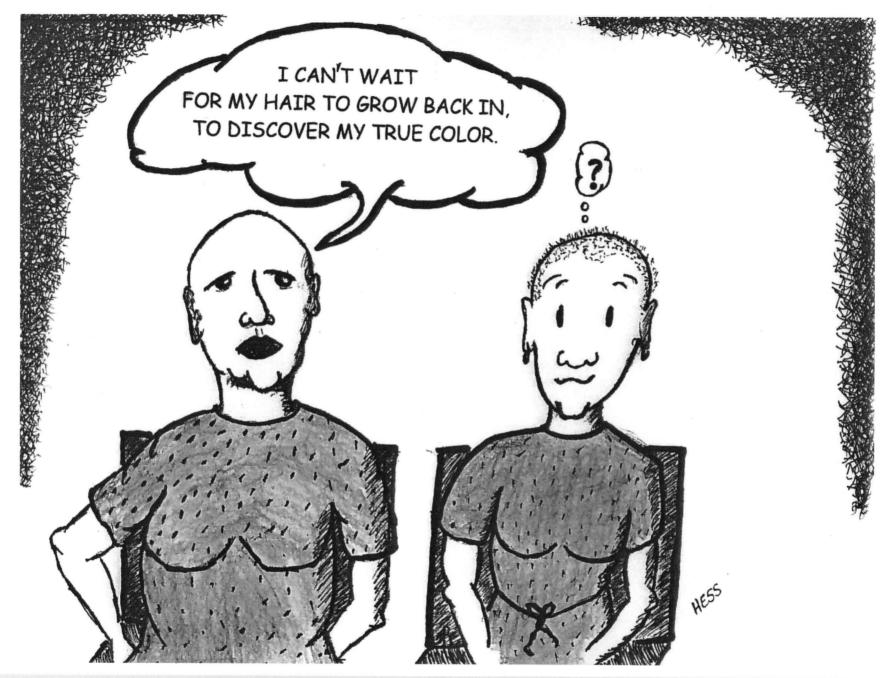

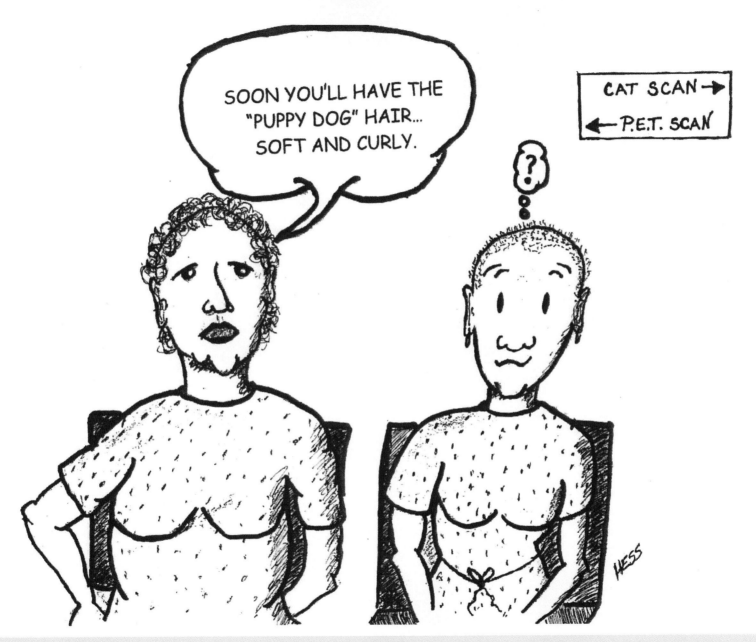

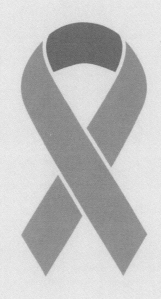

PART 7

Some Good Thoughts

67

AN EMOTIONAL JOURNEY: HUMOR AND HOPE THROUGH BREAST CANCER

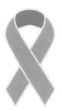

Your doctor informs you that you are "cancer free." What a day to celebrate! The difficulty you just went through now helps you to see the enhanced beauty of the good within your lives today. You may not mean to, but you change, and your family sees it. You say, "I am a survivor."

Your family thinks you are a superhero. Now you take the time to notice the simple things of life that nature provides us and realize you can be a helping hand or an emotional support to others while they are on their journey, no matter the type of cancer they might have.

Let's find some understanding and humor of your emotions on this journey...

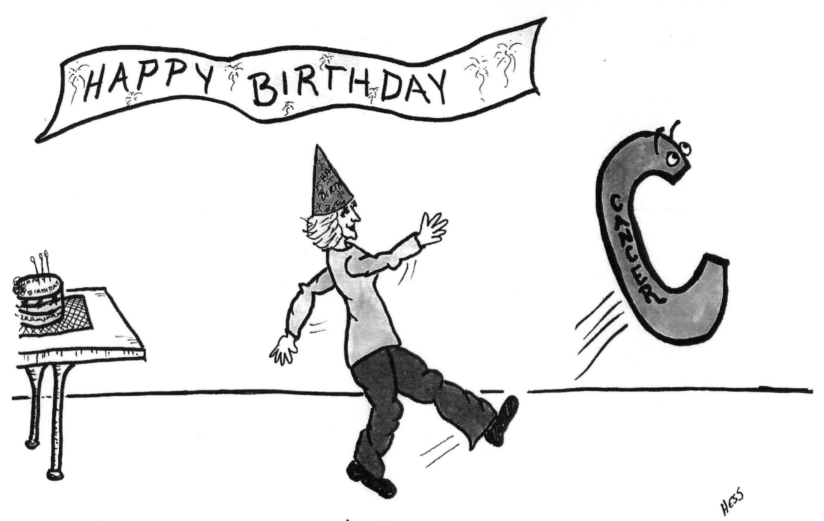

IT'S MY BIRTHDAY!!
AND WITH EACH ONE, THAT MEANS
I AM KICKING YOUR BUTT!

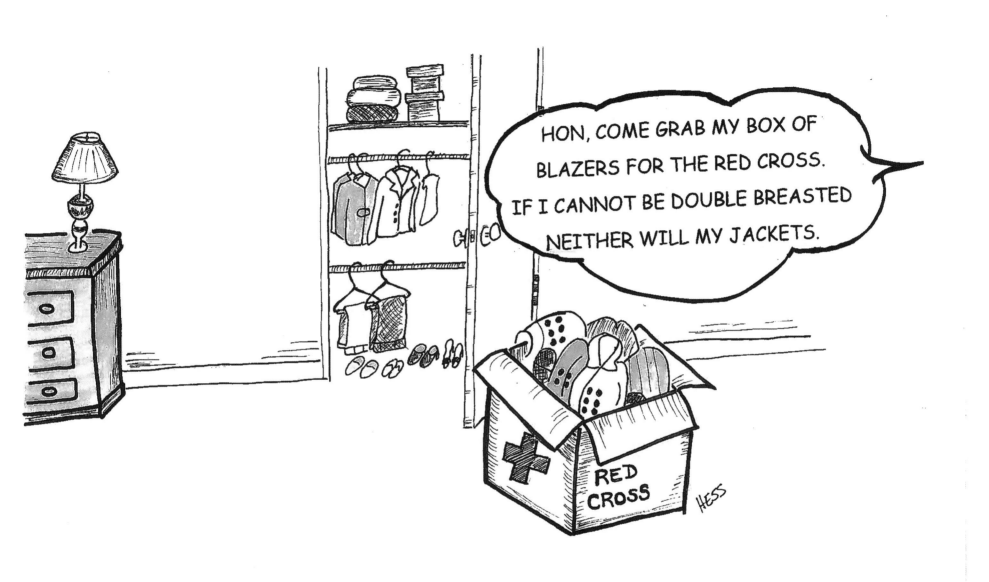

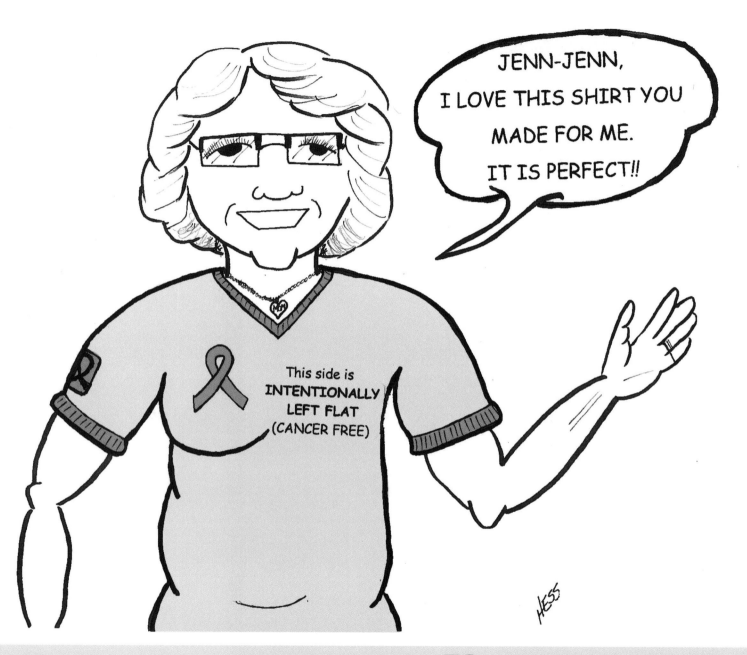

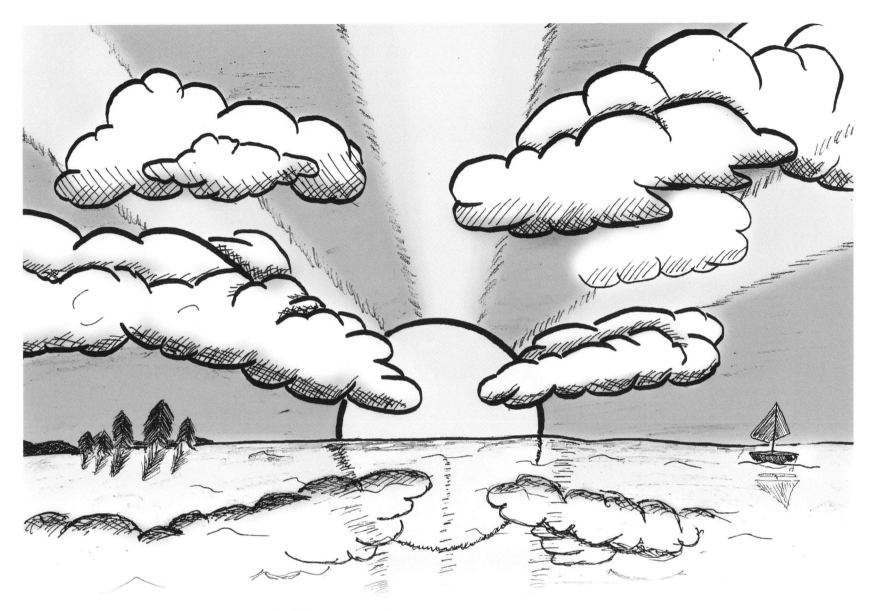

YOU NEED SOME CLOUDS TO REFLECT THE
BEAUTY OF A SUNSET.

HOPE

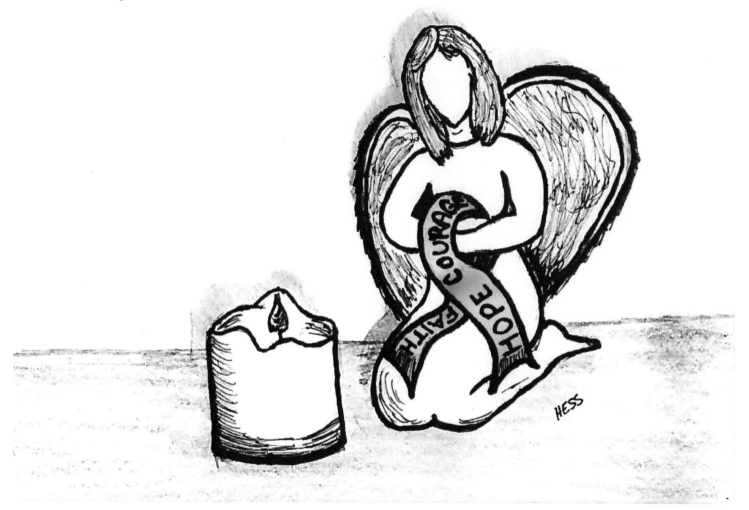

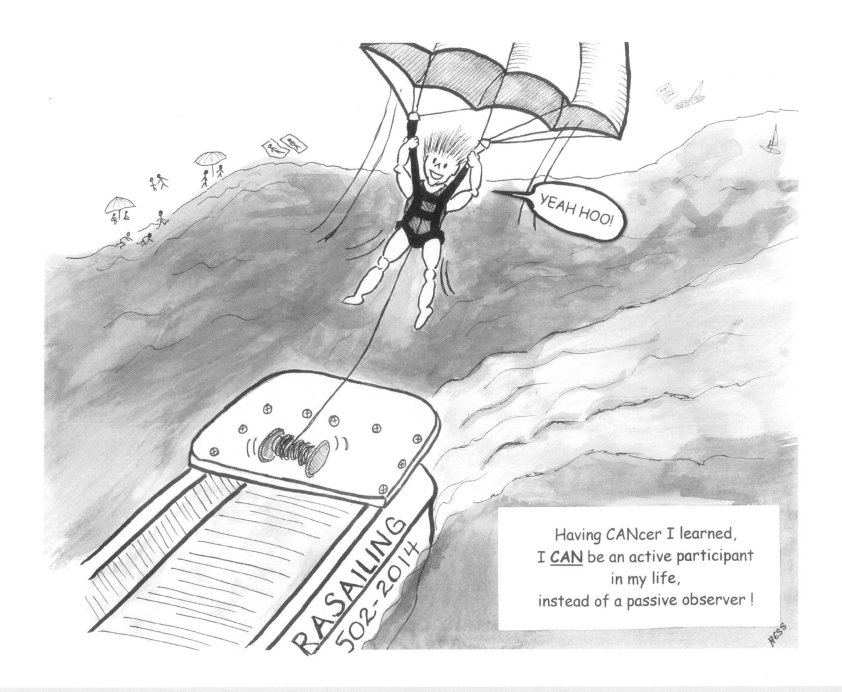

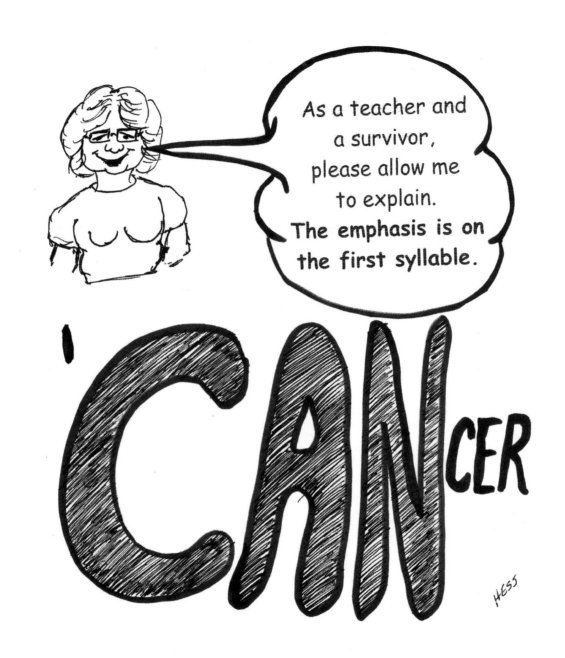

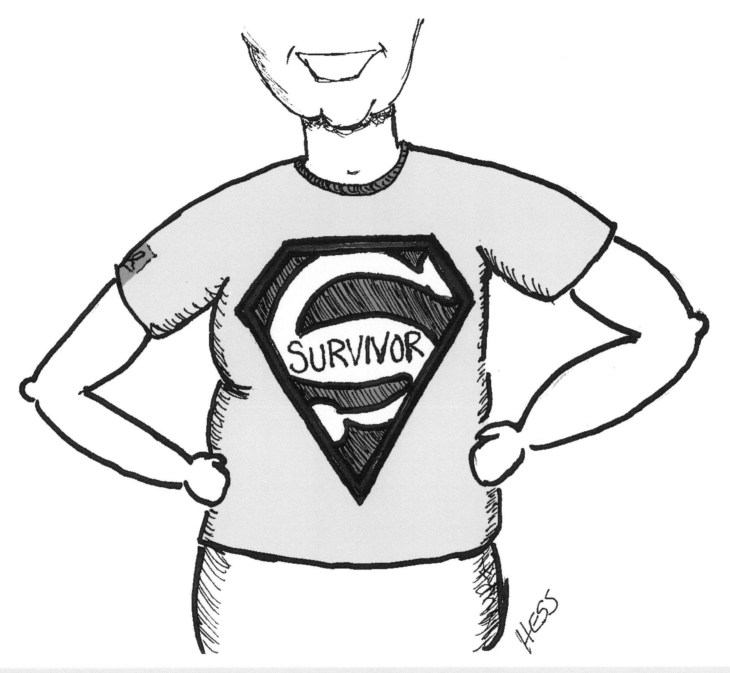

Page 16 Answers:

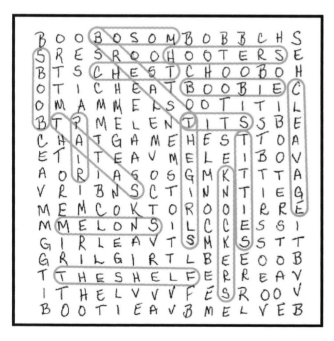

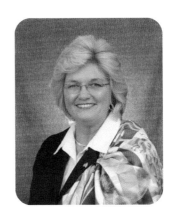

About the Author

Heather J. Rose-Fiorentino is one of nine in her family who have battled cancer. When her mother was stricken with a very aggressive cancer, she showed everyone how to live with cancer, with grace, a sense of humor, and a strong faith.

This strong role model and nine family members fighting a battle with cancer caused the rest of the family to understand it was when, not if they get cancer. So as an educator, Heather drew each situation in a journal of her battle (there were earlier cartoons of her mother's journey). With her family and friends' support, this book was produced after her second bout with cancer. Hess is a family nickname for Heather and she uses it as a pen name.

Heather's husband of thirty-three years, Joe, was a major support along with her children. Her daughter, Jennifer, was able to take her to some appointments, providing comfort and laughter, even on the day of surgery.

Now retired, Heather supports others as they fight cancer. Hoping to inspire and provide smiles during some of their rough days, Heather continues to draw cartoons, putting her unique twist on these fearful situations. Heather is working on her third book to inspire and provide hope and encouragement to others like her mother did years ago.

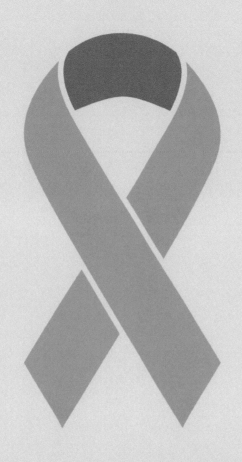

I hope this book gives you a different perspective and a better understanding, with a touch of humor, of your emotions while on your journey.

May God bless you!!